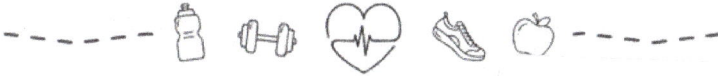

LOVE YOUR BODY

Unlock the Secrets to Reinvent Your Life, Change Your Body, and Improve Your Mind

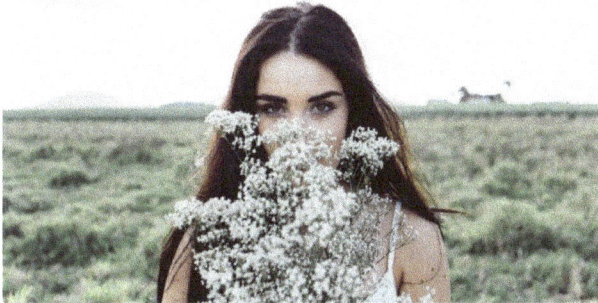

Dr. Gillian Keys Pomroy,
Dr. Anna Bernardi

THANK YOU FOR
PURCHASING THIS BOOK!

Table of Contents

Introduction:

Your Beginner's Guide to a Better Life

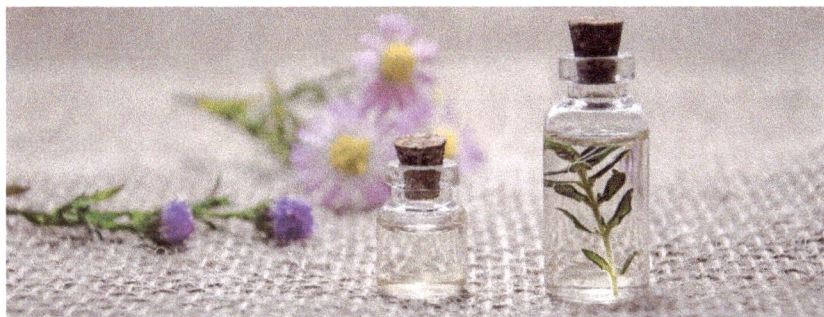

We all wish for a better life. But the question is, how do you achieve it?

The best way to do this is to start working towards the life you dream of having. The fact is, nothing will happen if you just sit there dreaming of what could be but not really do anything about it. There's no time like the present to start loving yourself more and working hard to improve yourself from within.

The good news is that you're reading this book right now and it's the perfect guide to help motivate you to love the body you're in. This book also aims to encourage further improvement by following a healthy diet and learning how to take care of yourself. If you want your life to become better, you need to start with yourself. Unless you feel happy, motivated, and confident in yourself, you might find it extremely challenging to go for the other things you truly want to achieve.

In this book, you'll learn all about how you can start improving your life by starting with yourself. With that being said, let's begin!

Chapter 1:

Clean Eating

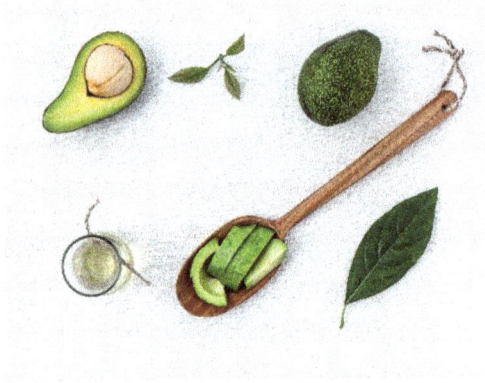

Essentially, clean eating is a diet—a specific way of eating. But you can also see it as a kind of lifestyle which helps improve your overall health and well-being. Simple as this diet is, clean eating involves a couple of key principles. These principles align with the basic principles of any healthy diet:

- **Choose real foods**

  This is the most common basic principle of healthy eating. If you want to start clean eating, then you must try to avoid refined or processed foods. Instead, opt for real foods which you either eat raw or which you can use to create healthy and tasty dishes. Often, the reason people go for packaged foods is convenience. This may be okay sometimes, but you can still go for products which contain real foods without artificial ingredients.

- **Eat for the purpose of nourishment**

  It's important for you to eat balanced, healthy meals and snacks regularly. Make sure these are nourishing and you don't rush through your meals. If possible, eat home-cooked meals, whether you cook them yourself or someone else in your home cooks them for you. Even if you go to work or you plan to travel, you can bring along packed home-cooked meals to avoid purchasing those "convenient" but usually unhealthy options.

- **Try to consume more plant-based food sources**

  When choosing what foods to eat, try to add more fruits and vegetables on your plate. The great thing about plant-based food sources is that you can get all the vitamins, minerals, and nutrients you need from them. For instance, we all need protein, right? You don't just have to get your protein from meat. There are a lot of plant-based food sources which contain protein such as whole grains, lentils, peas, beans, and much more.

- **Limit or avoid meat as much as possible**

  More and more studies have shown that limiting or avoiding meat is beneficial for overall health. Although clean eating doesn't require you to become a vegan or vegetarian, cutting back on your meat consumption can improve your health. You may have meat on occasion, but it's best to make plant-based foods the staple in your diet.

- **Limit added sugar**

  Unfortunately, a lot of people eat foods which are high in added sugars and this is never a good thing. If you want to clean up your eating habits, you may want to limit those common sweet treats such as baked goods, candy, soda, and the like. You may also want to check the sugar content of any "health foods" you plan to buy as these may contain added sugars too. This is why it's better to go for whole foods because you won't have to worry about any hidden ingredients.

- **Cut back on sodium**

  Sugar isn't the only issue when it comes to the foods we eat. Most people consume far more sodium than we actually need. If you want to limit your sodium intake, avoiding processed foods is an important step because these products typically contain high amounts of sodium. Although you can use salt in clean eating recipes, make sure to use this ingredient sparingly. Add it to bring out the flavors of your foods, not as the main flavor of your food.

- **Clean up your lifestyle**

  Part of clean eating is also adopting a cleaner lifestyle. Aside from eating the right foods, you should also get enough physical activity or exercise, get enough sleep each night, and learn how to manage stress properly. Also, connect with the people in your life. Talk to them, laugh with them, take a walk with them, and more. All of these will help you become a happier, healthier, and cleaner person.

- **It's about the environment too**

  The more people start clean eating, the more our planet will benefit. If more of us consume plant-based sources, this can help reduce the demand of the animal agricultural industry which, unfortunately, has a lot of negative effects on the environment. So, you can think about it this way: clean eating doesn't just have a positive impact on your life, it also has a positive impact on the planet.

The Health Benefits of Following a Healthy, Well-Balanced Diet

Now that you know more about clean eating, let's focus on the benefits of following such a diet. Following a healthy, clean diet means that you eat a lot of colorful fruits and veggies along with lean proteins, whole grains, starches, and good fats. It also means that you avoid foods which contain high amounts of unhealthy fats, sugar, and salt. Clean eating is an excellent diet and lifestyle because it provides you with these health benefits:

- **Weight loss**

   This is one thing a lot of people seem to be struggling with and it also happens to be one of the main frustrations of people all over the world. Although you may follow different kinds of diets, you just can't seem to shed those unwanted pounds! This may be because you're not following the diet properly or the type of diet you're following isn't suitable for your body.

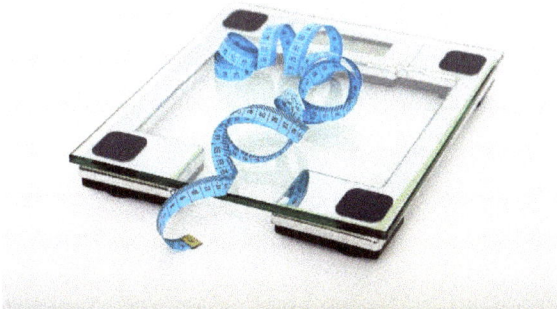

   When you follow a healthy, well-balanced diet, it can help you reach your weight-loss goals. Aside from this, losing weight may also help in reducing the risk of developing chronic health conditions.

- **Reduced risk of developing cancer**

  Consuming too many processed and refined foods may lead to different types of health conditions which may increase your risk of developing certain cancers. But if you go for whole, healthy foods, this may help reduce the risk. In fact, there are a lot of fruits, vegetables, and plant-based food sources which can even help protect you against these life-threatening conditions.

- **It helps in the management of diabetes**

  Clean eating allows people who suffer from diabetes to manage their levels of blood glucose, maintain healthy levels of cholesterol and blood pressure, and delay or prevent the complications that usually accompany this condition.

- **It promotes the health of the heart**

  Heart disease is a very common condition all around the world. According to research, different kinds of heart disease can be avoided by making changes in your lifestyle, such as eating healthier foods and having enough exercise or physical activity. Clean eating is the perfect diet to promote the health of the heart. So, if you already have heart disease or you are at high risk of developing the condition, this diet can be very beneficial for you.

- **It strengthens the bones and teeth**

  This is another excellent benefit of clean eating. As you follow a healthy and balanced diet, you're able to get enough of the essential nutrients each day. Nutrients such as magnesium and calcium are commonly found in plants and are essential for the strength of our teeth and bones. These nutrients also help prevent the development of osteoarthritis and osteoporosis later in life.

- **It may improve your mood**

  Many recent studies are finding a close relationship between our mood and our diet. For instance, diets that have a high glycemic level may increase the risk of developing the symptoms of depression. But if you follow a diet composed mainly of whole foods, you won't have to worry about this. Also, the more your diet makes you feel strong and healthy, the happier you will become.

- **It helps maintain the health of the brain to improve cognitive functions**

  Eating healthy foods helps maintain the health of your brain. This is very important since the brain oversees all the processes and functions of your body. Clean eating may help prevent cognitive decline so you may want to consider it if you want your mind to function well as you grow older.

- **It promotes gut health**

  Our gut is host to an entire ecosystem of bacteria, some of which are good while others are bad. A healthy diet promotes the health of our gut since the foods you eat are also the foods which nourish the good bacteria. This helps strengthen your immune system in order to reduce the risk of developing different kinds of illnesses and diseases.

- **It helps you get a good night sleep each night**

  Following a healthy diet may also help you sleep better each night. Most of the time, our sleeping patterns get disrupted by certain factors, such as drinking alcohol, obesity, and an unhealthy diet. When you clean up your life by eliminating these, you will be able to get enough rest to keep you healthy and strong.

The Most Common Issues People Have with Food and How to Overcome Them

Although food is one of our basic needs, a lot of us struggle with it. In the past, people didn't have a lot of options, so they ate similar things. However, currently there are endless selections of fresh produce, whole foods, processed foods, refined foods, and more. So, it can be overwhelming to follow just one diet and keep things simple.

Apart from finding it a challenge to eat healthy foods as opposed to the scrumptious but unhealthy options we are so used to eating, some people also succumb to a number of common issues with food. The sad thing with these issues is that overcoming them can seem like an impossible task, especially when you don't know how to do this or where to start. If all this seems familiar to you, then you may be suffering from one type of food issue or another. To help you overcome whatever it is you're dealing with, let's look at these common issues and how to deal with them:

1. **Over-eating**

    When it comes to eating, or rather, when it's time to stop eating, a lot of people struggle with self-control. Consuming too many calories each day or eating too much each meal or in a single sitting are very common habits which are very challenging to break. Unfortunately, overeating leads to weight gain which increases your risk of developing chronic diseases.

    Also, overeating prevents you from reaching your fitness, wellness, and health goals. If you tend to overeat, you may find it difficult to start a clean eating lifestyle as well. If you want to overcome this, here are some tips which may help you:

- Avoid doing other things while you're eating so you can focus more on what you put in your mouth and when you already feel full.
- Learn about your food weaknesses so you can take steps in limiting or restricting your intake.
- Don't restrict yourself too much, especially in terms of your favorite foods.
- Try "volumetrics," where you fill up with high-fiber, low-calorie foods right before eating your regular meals.
- Avoid eating meals and snacks directly from the containers so you can control your portions.
- Learn how to deal with stress instead of eating through it.
- Eat a lot of foods which are rich in fiber.
- Don't skip meals.
- Dine frequently with people who share the same health and food goals as you.
- Eat slowly and chew your food thoroughly.
- Try to limit your consumption of alcoholic beverages.
- Give meal planning a try.
- Drink water instead of sugary beverages.
- Don't focus on "dieting." Instead, focus on following a healthy lifestyle.
- Set goals and stick with them.

2. Binge Eating

Binge Eating Disorder or BED is one of the most common eating disorders in America and it's a very challenging issue to overcome. People who suffer from this condition tend to eat an unusually large amount of food even if they don't feel hungry. They then feel ashamed and guilty after, making this condition damaging to physical, mental, and emotional health. If you want to overcome your tendency to binge eat, try these strategies:

- Don't deprive yourself by convincing yourself that you should follow a strict diet.
- Make sure that you eat meals regularly.
- Learn "mindful eating," which makes you more aware of what you're eating and how you feel while you're eating.
- Drink enough water to stay hydrated.
- Give yoga a try.
- Remember that fiber-rich foods are your friend.
- Clean out your home, especially your kitchen.
- Consider starting your own exercise routine.
- Never skip breakfast.
- Make sure that you get enough sleep each night.
- Try keeping a food journal (more on this later).
- Talk about your issue with someone whom you know can help you deal with it.

3. Under-eating

On the other side of the spectrum, there are some people who don't eat enough each day. In fact, they eat such small amounts of food that they are starting to damage their health as well. A lot of people who end up under-eating are usually those who try to cut their caloric intake to lose weight. But not eating isn't the answer! If you find yourself struggling with this problem, here are some tips which may help you:

- Instead of skipping meals, learn how to make healthier food choices to help you reach your food goal.
- Don't focus too much on what you need to do to lose weight.

- o Focus on following a healthy lifestyle and a clean diet in order to make yourself feel better.
- o Keeping a food diary or journal may also be helpful with this issue.
- o If you think you need help, consult with a profes-sional.

Chapter 2:

Finding Physical and Mental Energy

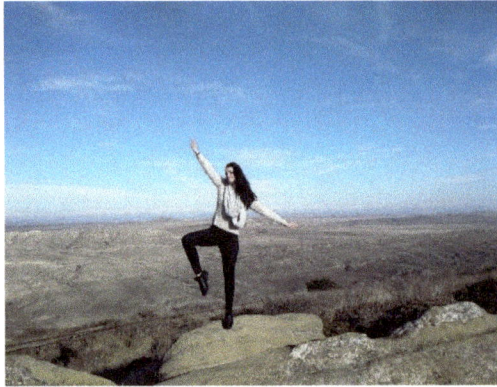

After cleaning up your diet and lifestyle, it's time to find physical and mental energy to keep you going. If you want to be the best version of yourself, someone you love and accept completely, there are a lot of things you must do. To acquire the energy you need, movement and physical activity are key.

Often, health experts claim that exercising for at least half an hour, five time each week can already help you become a healthier individual. But exercising regularly comes with benefits that go beyond having a healthy body, it also helps improve your mental health. Let's look at some of these benefits:

1. **The physical benefits of exercise**

   o It helps your body burn fat at a much faster rate, thus leading to significant weight loss.
   o It helps strengthen the body by building muscle tone and mass.
   o It helps raise energy levels to improve your agility and performance.

- It helps keep the shape of the body protected as it increases overall muscle strength and flexibility.
- It helps enhance neuromuscular coordination while also developing a stronger skeletal structure.
- It helps make the immune system stronger while improving the gastrointestinal and digestive processes.
- It helps in the management of different disorders such as hypertension, diabetes, cardiovascular disease, and more.
- It helps lower the risk of developing some cancer types.

2. The mental benefits of exercise

- It improves concentration and memory.
- It stimulates endorphin production to help calm the mind as well as reduce the effects of depression and stress.
- It enhances mental agility and self-confidence.
- It plays an important role in controlling discontent thus making it crucial for the process of anger management.
- It promotes high-quality sleep which is crucial for the health and normal functioning of the brain.

How to Remain Physically Active

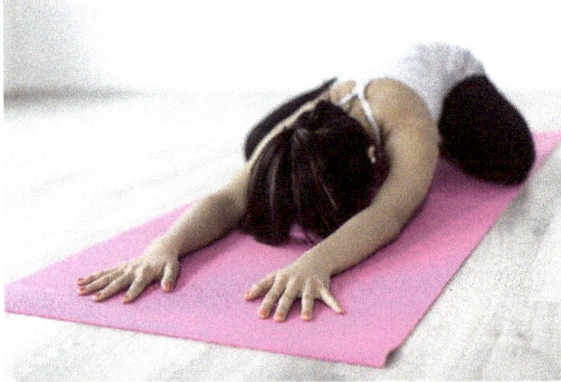

If you want to start living a healthier lifestyle, one of the best things that you can do is to start your own fitness program to ensure that you always remain physically active. This doesn't necessarily mean that you should go to the gym and spend your time there. When it comes to physical activity, go at your own pace. You don't have to be an athlete to become healthy.

In fact, if you can find a physical activity which you really enjoy and which makes you feel good, there's a higher chance that you'll stick with it. Here are some steps for you to follow in order to start your own customized fitness program:

- **Assess your own level of fitness**

  Think about yourself right now and try to assess your fitness level. Do you engage in a lot of physical activities each day or do you spend most of your time sitting down while working? This is the first thing you must do.

  Part of the assessment is to record your baseline fitness scores to have a benchmark to use when you're measuring your progress. In order to get these baseline scores, record the following:

  - Your resting pulse rate.

- Your pulse rate right after you have walked one mile.
- How long it takes you to walk one mile.
- How long it takes you to run one and a half miles.
- How many standard push-ups, modified push-ups or half sit-ups you can do at one time.
- The distance you can reach when you stretch your arm forward while sitting on the floor.
- The circumference of your waist.
- Your BMI or body mass index.

- **Design your custom fitness program**

  Saying that you'll exercise daily is a lot easier than actually doing it. If you want to solidify your resolve, the best thing you can do is come up with a plan for your fitness program. When you design this program, here are some pointers to keep in mind:

  - Think about the fitness goals you want to achieve. Setting these goals and making them clear helps you keep track of your progress while staying motivated.
  - Create a balanced fitness program. Start off slowly and gradually increase the frequency and intensity of your physical activity. This helps your body adjust to this new routine.
  - Try to find time for physical activity in your daily routine. Although this may be challenging, you can look schedule exercise times as you would schedule your other appointments. If you think it will help, pair your exercise activities with activities you enjoy. For instance, you can take a walk while listening to music, jog on a treadmill while watching your favorite shows, and so on.

- Vary your physical activities and exercises. This makes it more effective as opposed to doing the same thing repeatedly.
- Make recovery part of your plan. It's never a good idea to push your body too hard as you might get injured or you might start experiencing aches and pains. When you create your fitness program, don't forget to include relaxation and recovery.

- **Assemble all the equipment you need**

  The types of equipment you would assemble depends on the types of physical activities you plan to incorporate into your daily routine. For instance, if you love running or power walking, you must have the right shoes for this. If you don't own a good pair of running or power walking shoes, this is the first thing you must get for yourself.

  If you want to invest in various exercise equipment, make sure to choose those that are fun and easy to use, as well as practical. You can try out the different equipment at fitness centers before you purchase your own personal exercise equipment.

  Finally, you may also want to download a good fitness or activity tracking app on your smartphone to help you with your physical activities. Such apps are very useful because you can keep track of your progress on them. The more you see improvement, the more motivated you will be.

- **Get started!**

  After all the planning, it's time to get started. Remember that this is something you will be doing long-term in order to improve your physical, emotional, and mental health. Although it may seem challenging at first, keep with it, especially if you want to enjoy all the benefits. Here are some things to keep in mind as you start your new fitness program:

- o Start slowly then gradually build up your routine when you think you're ready for more.
- o If you feel like you can't handle the routine at the beginning, break up the activities.
- o When it comes to thinking of exercises and physical activities, be as creative as possible to make it more fun and motivating.
- o Listen to and be aware of your body. If you're feeling dizziness, pain, and other unusual symptoms, rest for a while.
- o Don't take your fitness program too seriously. If you feel like you're pushing yourself too hard, take a break and relax.

- **Keep track of your progress**

  Finally, don't forget to keep track of your progress. You can do this by keeping a fitness journal, a digital diary, or by using a fitness app. It doesn't matter how you monitor your progress; the important thing is that you always keep track of how you're doing.

Motivating Yourself to Keep Going

Now that you have your own custom fitness program, the next thing to do is to make sure that you stick to it. Often, people feel very enthusiastic at the beginning, but they soon lose their motivation to keep going, especially when they don't see or feel immediate results. Nobody said that change is easy. But if you put in the time and effort, the time will come when you will see the fruits of your labor.

No matter how driven you are to become more physically active, you won't start feeling the benefits until you start moving and you learn how to motivate yourself to continue with what you've planned each day. Motivation is a huge part of this process. But how do you keep yourself motivated?

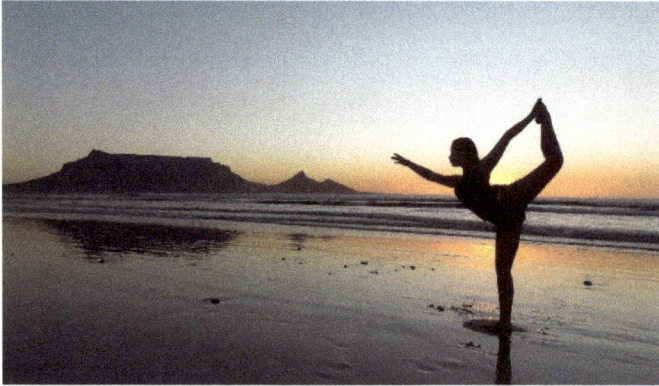

Here are some helpful suggestions for you:

- **Invite someone to take this fitness journey with you**

  Most of the time, we feel more motivated when we're exercising or doing a fun physical activity with a friend. When you're able to find a buddy to workout with, you can encourage and support each other to stick with your plans until you've reached your goals and beyond.

- **Join a fitness club**

  For some people, they feel more motivated when they're part of a group. If you're this type of person, then the best thing for you to do is join a fitness class, a fitness club, or a fitness group. This may help motivate you and it can also help you meet new friends.

- **Start a competition... with yourself**

  This suggestion is especially useful if you are a competitive person. When you compete with yourself, it's like you are pushing yourself to become better each time. Of course, don't forget to listen to your body. You may be so intent on beating your own record that you end up compromising your health. Just as when you're competing with others, you should engage in a healthy sort of competition with yourself.

- **Join actual competitions**

There are different kinds of fitness competitions you can attend, such as marathons. These are usually held within the community and they're usually a lot of fun! Again, apart from being able to add to your physical activities, you will be able to meet a lot of like-minded people when you join these kinds of competitions.

- **Listen to music**

Music can be a powerful motivator. When you're feeling down or lazy, try playing some upbeat dance music, preferably those which you really love. Soon, you'll find yourself feeling more energized. You can also turn the TV on while you're doing your physical activity if you think that it will help. You can do push-ups or sit-ups while watching your shows. Pairing your exercise with a fun activity makes it easier to get through it.

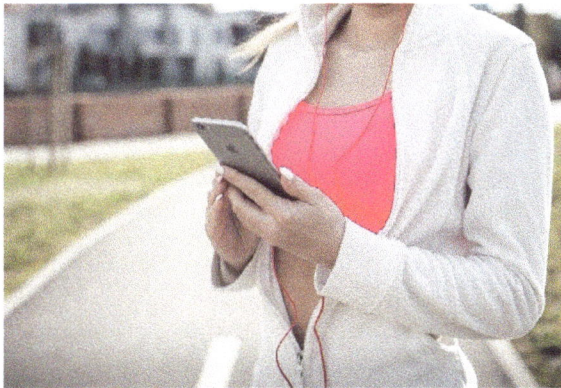

- **Read about people who have succeeded**

  Another thing you can do to remain motivated is to read some inspiring success stories. If you're feeling particularly overwhelmed or challenged, go online and search for these stories. There are a lot of them out there. So many people have faced the same challenges at the beginning of their journeys. The important thing is that you want to make a change, so do everything that you can to keep yourself motivated.

- **Never push yourself**

  Although this has already been mentioned, it's worth mentioning again. Yes, you want to improve your life by becoming more physically active. But pushing yourself too hard isn't the way to go. If you start feeling discomfort or pain, stop and allow your body to recover. And when you give yourself time off, don't feel guilty about it. Keep in mind that you're trying to learn how to love and accept yourself more. So, do things at your own pace and this will make you feel more inspired in the long-run.

Chapter 3:
Getting Started

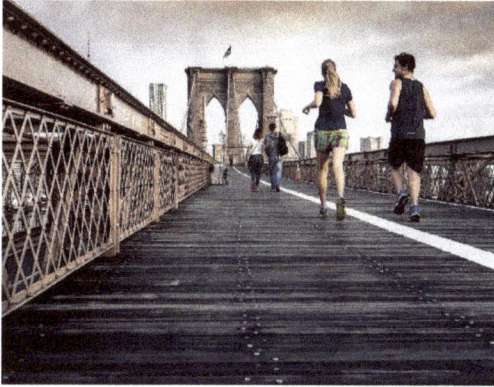

Are you feeling more positive towards yourself yet?

If not, don't worry, we're just getting started. Anyone who plans to improve their life must commit to it. It's not just about saying that you want things to get better, it's more about doing something to initiate that change. For some people, loving themselves isn't an easy task, especially when they lived most of their lives being negative and cynical.

Happiness is a choice and the more you work on having it, the easier this choice becomes. Now, let's help you get started. Although you may not feel happy or satisfied with your body right now, this doesn't mean that you can be. Come up with a plan with achievable and actionable steps to help point you in the right direction. To make it easier for you, let's look at some easy steps to help you with getting started.

Setting Goals

No matter what kind of change you plan to make in your life, the first thing you must do is set goals for yourself. It's very difficult to think of steps to make you love your body more when you don't have concrete goals to look forward to. It's not as simple as waking up tomorrow and telling yourself that "I will love the body I have."

Sure, this might make you feel better for some time, but sooner or later reality kicks in and you're left having to deal with everything else in your life. Then you forget what you told yourself and each time a challenging situation comes up, you go right back to how you previously saw, felt, and thought about yourself.

Setting goals makes it easier for you to plan for what you want and think of steps on how you can get there. The best part is that you don't even have to think of huge or difficult goals! As a matter of fact, it's much more effective to come up with one long-term goal and a few short-term goals to keep you motivated along the way. To illustrate this better, here's an example:

Let's say you feel unhappy or unsatisfied with your body because you feel like you're overweight. This is one of the most common reasons why people don't love their bodies. In this case, you can make a list of goals, such as:

- **Long-term goal: Reach your target weight.**

- **Short-term goals:**
    - Come up with a fitness plan.
    - Learn about the different kinds of healthy diets and lifestyles.
    - Determine which diet or lifestyle suits you.
    - Make a plan to follow the diet and lifestyle you've chosen.

These are only a few examples of goals you can set for yourself. As you can see, you would have one long-term goal and a number of short-term goals which will help you move towards your main goal bit by bit. Come up with a list of your own and use that for the next step.

Having a Plan

After you've decided on your goals, it's time to come up with a plan to achieve each of them. This is an effective way for you to have a guide for what you need to do. Anytime you feel overwhelmed, confused, or lost, all you have to do is go back to the plan you've made and see what comes next.

Although some people don't like making plans, this is actually a very helpful way to ensure that you will reach the goals you've set for yourself. Take some time to reflect on these goals and think about how you will be able to reach them. You don't have to treat this step like a chore or something too difficult. Since you'll be the one thinking of the steps, you can make them as simple or as complex as you want them to be.

Using the same example from the first step, let's try to come up with a plan for one of the short-term goals we've mentioned:

- **Goal: Learn about the different kinds of healthy diets and lifestyles**

  There are so many types of diets out there and they all come with their own advantages and disadvantages. Before you can choose which one suits you the most, you need to learn all about them. Here are some steps for you to do this:

  - Go online and search for a list of different kinds of diets. Try to find a website that provides a list along with a short description to give you a better idea of what they're all about.

- o Make your own list of the diets which seem appealing to you. You should choose 3-5 diets that you think you will be able to follow.
- o Now, learn about these diets individually. As you learn more about them, you will have a better idea of what each diet involves and whether it's right for you.
- o Narrow down your options to 2-3.

Since your goal here was merely to learn about the different diets, when you reach this step, you're done! The simpler your short-term goals are, the more effortlessly you will be able to achieve them. This is important, especially at the beginning, as it will keep you motivated to move on to the next step until you've finally reached your main goal.

Being Realistic

From the time you decide to embark on a journey towards becoming more loving and happier with your body, you must always remember to be realistic. There's nothing more disheartening than trying to achieve idealistic or impractical goals. Setting such goals would be like setting yourself up to fail, so you may want to rethink your strategy.

Being realistic is easy. All you have to do is think about what you want and what you can do about it. If you don't love your body, reflect on why that is. Are you really unhappy or do you simply feel despondent whenever you try to compare yourself with other people? Are you unhappy because your size doesn't allow you to be as mobile or as agile as you want to be? Are you unhappy because you always feel physically tired and weak? Or are you unhappy because you're not as fit as you want to be?

There are many reasons why people are able to love others with all their heart but aren't able to give themselves that same degree of affection. Whatever your reason is, it's time to start changing this. Because when you think about it, you really won't be able to love others completely unless you learn to love yourself as well.

Going back to being realistic, this mainly applies to the goals you will set for yourself. Go back to the list of goals you created and try to determine if they're realistic enough. Think about your own skills, capabilities, and even the time you have to take the steps to reach those goals. If you think that the goals you've listed down are realistic and doable, that's great! If not, you may have to make a few changes to them in order to make it easier for you to achieve them all.

Knowing How to Adjust as You Go

Speaking of making changes, this is an important part of this last step for getting started. Even though you've spent a lot of time and effort into coming up with your goals and your plans for these goals, that doesn't mean that they're written in stone. This means that if you happen to encounter a challenge along the way, you must also know how to adjust as you go.

There's nothing wrong with challenges and failures. As long as you try your best to overcome them, these hardships will make you stronger and more resilient. In cases where you find it difficult to reach one of your goals, whether it be short-term or long-term, don't be discouraged. Instead, try to think of a way to make an adjustment to your plan or to the goal you have set.

Maybe you had just set a goal which is too difficult for you to achieve at that moment. In that case, what you can do is break down the goal into two or three parts, making it easier to achieve. If the trouble lies in one of the steps in your plan, then adjustment that too. Learn how to be flexible when it comes to achieving your goals. As long as you're working towards these goals, it doesn't really matter how you do it.

Also, learning how to adjust as you go helps you learn to be more accepting of yourself. Instead of feeling bad or berating yourself for not being able to conquer challenges, you simply pick yourself up and find a way to deal with the situation. In doing this, you'll see how easy it is to become more loving and happier with yourself too.

Chapter 4:
The Dos and Don'ts of Loving Your Body

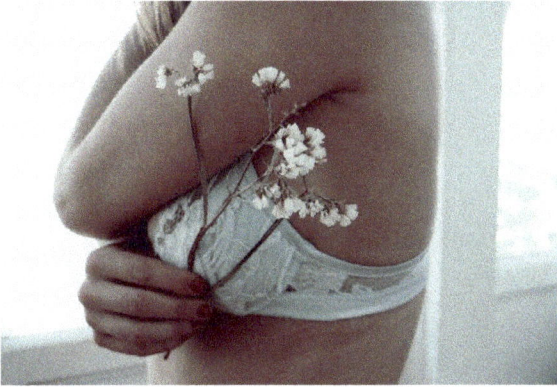

Loving your body is easy. That is, if you know what it really means and what it entails. Think about how you feel about your body right now. Are you happy with it? Is there something which you'd like to change about it? Are you comfortable with your own body?

Some people may say that they love their body but they're not confident about it at all. So, they hide behind layers of clothing while calling this their style. Then when they're on their own and they get the chance to see or feel their body, they feel a sense of discontent or a yearning for something better.

If this situation sounds familiar to you, then maybe you're not happy with your body. Of course, this doesn't mean that fit or slim people are the only ones who are happy with the bodies they have. Sometimes, even the people that others envy want something else. This is the biggest issue when it comes to learning how to love your body. It's not just about achieving the "perfect" body, it's more about accepting the body you have and being comfortable in your own skin.

There are some do's and don'ts that come with loving your body. Although these are general suggestions, you should still try to find what works for you personally. Remember that you are unique, and this means that what may work well for someone else might not work for you in the same way. Therefore, you may have to try a few things and see which ones are suitable for you and which ones you can do without.

Make Sure to DO These Things

We should all take care of our bodies every day. It doesn't matter whether you're completely happy with it or there are things which you would like to change, taking care of your body is an important part of loving yourself. The most basic ways to do this are to learn how to reduce stress in your life, eat healthy foods, exercise regularly, and take a break when you need to.

We all know that taking care of yourself is important. But, doing this isn't easy for everyone. Most people are too busy with the other aspects of their lives to practice self-care. Often, self-care becomes the last thing on our list of priorities. Unfortunately, over time, this can start taking a toll on your body. But loving yourself means that you care for yourself too. Here are some things you should start doing as part of your quest for self-love:

- **DO make adequate sleep a part of your daily self-care regimen**

   Sleep is an essential part of our lives because it has a significant impact on how we feel both physically and emotionally. When you don't get enough sleep, you usually end up being cranky for the whole day. Aside from this, a lack of sleep can also increase your risk of developing a number of health issues.

You must make sure that you clock in enough hours of sleep each night. If your problem is not being able to fall asleep on time, then you may want to start a bedtime routine. Find ways to wind down before going to bed so your body knows when it's time to go to sleep.

Part of being able to fall asleep and stay asleep throughout the night is learning how to deal with and reduce stress in your life. If you're able to do this, you won't be troubled by issues which may hinder you from getting a good night's rest.

- **DO prioritize your gut health**

You may not be aware of it, but the health of your gut influences your overall well-being, health, and vitality. That's why it's important for you to make sure that you always have a healthy gut. A happy and healthy gut makes you a happy and healthy person which allows you to love and appreciate your body more.

- **DO eat right and exercise regularly**

We've already gone through the importance and benefits of these two things. No matter what kind of good change you want to happen in your life, it will always involve a healthy diet and regular exercise. This is because doing both ensures good health so that you will have the strength and motivation to do everything else.

- **DO prioritize yourself**

This doesn't mean that you should be selfish in a way that you don't value the other people in your life. It just means that you should start taking better care of yourself just as much as you take care of your partner, your parents or your children. Think about it, if you get sick or if you get to a point where you're so unhappy with yourself that you can't function normally, you're not the only one who will suffer. Make sure self-care is part of your daily routine. And if you need to take a break, do it!

- **DO spend some time outdoors**

  There's really nothing like getting a breath of fresh air. Have you ever seen how happy children are when they are playing outside? This is because they get to do a fun activity in an environment that makes them feel free. Try this out sometime. Take a short stroll around the neighborhood, read a book in your backyard or do something else which relaxes you out in the world. Doing this might even make you feel more connected with your body, your thoughts, and your emotions.

- **DO organize your life**

  Sometimes the problems in our life come from us not being organized enough. We often feel stressed or inadequate because we're not able to deal with things in an organized manner. Try to come up with a plan or a way to bring order into your life. Then you may discover that you actually have free time to do other things which you enjoy, and which make you feel good about yourself.

These are some suggestions for you to start your own self-care routine. There are so many other things you can do which can help you love yourself and your body more. Just as with setting goals and creating plans, find out which works for you and keep doing that.

The DON'TS to Avoid

Of course, if there are things you must do, there are also things which you should avoid. Loving your body doesn't mean that there are no limitations and that you can do no wrong. Self-care doesn't really have to be a time-consuming or challenging process. In fact, the more you do these practices, you may start learning to appreciate and enjoy them. Just make sure you avoid the following:

- **DON'T overdo it**

  Some people indulge in too much self-care and this isn't a good thing. Keep in mind that life is all about moderation and balance. Becoming truly appreciative and fulfilled means that you have to undergo stress and challenges at some point. Don't shy from experiences just because you're not sure about the outcomes and you don't want to feel stressed since you want to "take care of yourself." Never use your self-care practices as a reason to avoid things in life.

- **DON'T forget about the basics**

  What comes to mind when you hear the term "self-care?" These days, for a lot of people, this means going to spas, having massages, using fancy beauty products, and the like. But that isn't all there is. To love your body, never forget about the basics. Staying healthy can be as easy as drinking enough water, eating healthy and balanced meals, getting adequate sleep, and exercising regularly. Simple and basic as these steps are, they will always be highly effective.

- **DON'T spend too much money on your self-care practices**

  Although there's nothing wrong with spending money on yourself, you mustn't use your self-care practices as an excuse to spend too much money. For instance, if you see a cute item of clothing and when you tried it on, you discover that it looks great on you. If you don't normally spend a lot on clothing, this is the perfect time to splurge on yourself. In this example, you want the item and you need it too.

It is very different to splurge on a bunch of beauty products which claim that they can help improve a part of your body which, incidentally, is the part you feel fairly insecure about. Before spending money on anything, think about it first. This doesn't mean that you should micromanage yourself, it just means that you should be more practical when it comes to your self-care.

- **DON'T just depend on what TV or social media tells you**

Television and social media are both a blessing and a curse. Through these modern inventions, we can connect with the world in a way that the people in the past only dreamed of. Through television, we're able to learn more about the world and what's happening in it. Through social media, we're able to connect with others and be updated about their lives on a global scale.

At the same time, both TV and social media can have a negative impact on our lives, especially in terms of how we feel about our bodies and ourselves. All you see on TV and social media are "perfect people" leading perfect lives. Sometimes, they also encourage you to follow a certain lifestyle or a certain diet or even buy certain products so you can be just like them.

Realistically speaking, do you think simply buying something or following a diet will change your life in an instant? Obviously, the answer is no. But when you're feeling unhappy or vulnerable about your body, you tend to believe or *want* to believe everything you see and hear on TV and on social media.

As much as you can, try to avoid this. Don't rely on this information solely. Do your own research, talk to other people, and try to learn as much as you can about the things you want to do or buy before you make a choice. That way, you're prepared for all the consequences of your choice.

- **DON'T believe that "one size fits all"**

Finally, keep in mind that each person is unique. Self-care involves caring for yourself, not for anyone else. Although you may ask advice from other people or read about how you can care for yourself more effectively, it all boils down to you. You have to decide what's best for you, what makes you feel comfortable, and what makes you happy.

Chapter 5:

Shopping and Cooking

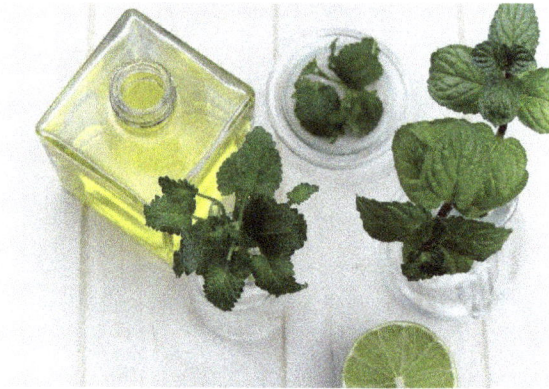

Changing your diet involves more than just ordering different kinds of dishes from restaurants. Since you will be eating most of your meals at home, you must also make changes in your shopping habits and in the way you cook your food.

An important part of loving your body is nourishing it properly. If the diet you're currently following includes a lot of processed, refined, and generally unhealthy options, it's time to start making a new list of foods to shop for. It's also time to start learning how to cook new dishes using those fresh, healthy ingredients you've bought.

The Importance of Cooking from Home Using Healthy Ingredients

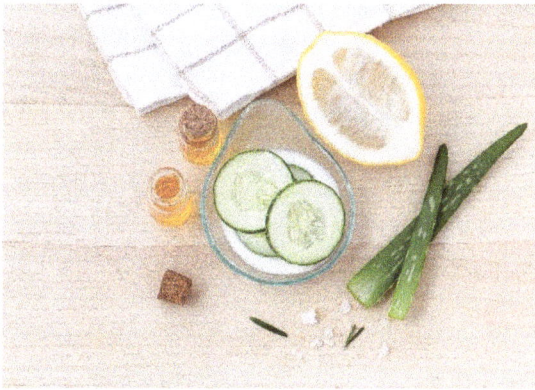

These days, we are so busy with our lives that cooking from home seems like such a chore. This is one of the reasons why most people choose to dine out with their families and friends. But this isn't recommended, especially when you're trying to make changes in your lifestyle. Dining out too frequently or indulging in convenient processed and pre-packaged foods won't help you become a healthier person. These options are also costly and unhealthy.

To keep up with your journey to self-improvement, you should try cooking from home more often. There are many benefits to doing this including:

- **It's healthier**

  Restaurants, fast food chains, and convenience stores may offer ready-made meals, but these are typically high in fats, carbohydrates, sugars, sodium, and calories. Often, they also have very low nutritional content. But if you cook your own food using fresh, whole ingredients you've purchased from your local grocery store, you will be able to get healthier and more nourishing meals.

- **You'll learn more about food**

  The more you cook from home, the more you will be able to learn about food. You'll learn that the food we eat isn't just something to fill your stomach. Food has the potential to inflict pain, cause illnesses, and heal as well. All these effects depend on the kind of food you eat, and you will learn more about this as you explore different kinds of ingredients and recipes.

- **It gives you a new appreciation for food**

  Physically preparing and cooking your own food leads to a new kind of appreciation for what you eat. As you chop, grate, fry, boil, and more, you're able to experience your foods with all your senses. This is very important, especially when it comes to mindful eating. The more aware you are of the food you eat, the more you'll be able to feel how the food affects you and whether this effect is positive or negative.

- **You can control the portions of the food you cook and eat**

  When you order food from restaurants, the dishes usually come in huge portion sizes. So, you can either eat everything on your plate or let the rest go to waste. Neither option is ideal. But when you cook your own food, you will be able to control the portions you put on your plate and whatever's leftover, you can store in your refrigerator for another day.

- **Helps you build healthier habits**

  Learning how to cook your meals from home is an excellent first step to jump-start your healthy diet and lifestyle. There are so many sources where you can find healthy recipes to whip up in your own kitchen. Over time, you will start seeing the value of following a healthier diet which, in turn, may motivate you to start other healthy habits.

- **Safety and cleanliness**

    When you purchase the ingredients yourself, prepare these ingredients, and cook them using your own kitchen utensils, you know that the food you eat is safe and clean. You don't have to worry about getting sick because of poor sanitation or unclean preparation.

- **You'll save a lot of money**

    Finally, cooking from home is also more economical. Rather than spending your money on fancy restaurants and unhealthy processed foods, use it to buy fresh ingredients. The great thing about these is that they are typically cheaper than prepared meals. Then once you get home, you can use these ingredients to whip up healthy and tasty meals.

The Importance of Meal Planning

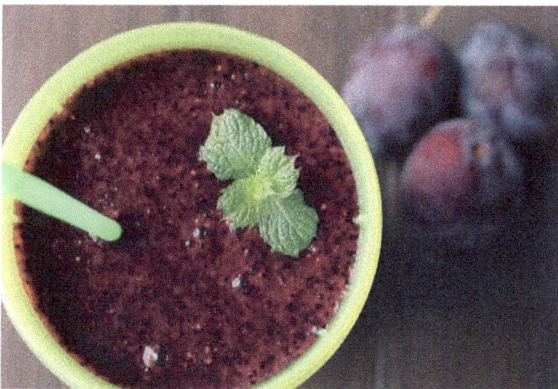

One of the biggest reasons why people don't want to cook their meals from home is that the process is quite time-consuming. When you compare cooking to ordering food from a restaurant, this is definitely true. But have you ever heard about meal planning?

Simply put, meal planning is when you set a specific schedule (usually one day each week) to plan, prepare, and cook your meals for the whole week. For instance, if you don't work on weekends, you may do your shopping on Saturday and your cooking on Sunday, or you may do both on one day. Then, you would store these meals in your freezer or refrigerator. Each day, you would simply heat up the meals you have prepared for breakfast, lunch, and dinner. It's as simple as that!

The great thing about meal planning is that it gives you total control over everything you eat at each meal and for each day. It starts with planning, then budgeting, shopping, preparing, and storing. Although this process may take some getting used to, the more you do it, the easier it gets.

Still not convinced? Here are some reasons that explain the advantages of meal planning:

- **You save time**

  This reason is very appealing, especially for those who always seem to be in a rush. We all have days off, right? Take some time out of those days off for meal planning. The time you spend for this process will allow you to have tasty, healthy, home-cooked meals every day for the rest of the week.

  This means that you won't have to cook your meals individually nor would you have to spend so much money ordering from restaurants. All you have to do is take the meals you have prepared from your refrigerator, heat them up if needed, and enjoy!

  Meal planning also saves you a lot of time at the grocery store. After you've planned your meals for the week, you would write down all the ingredients you need on your shopping list. As you enter the supermarket, you know exactly what you will buy, therefore, you won't spend so much time wandering around while you decide what to buy. And as long as you stick with your list, you won't end up buying unnecessary items that are a waste of money. It's definitely a win-win situation.

- **You eat healthier meals**

  Since meal planning involves cooking your meals from home, both processes share this same benefit. When you plan your meals, you have the freedom to make them as creative, tasty, and healthy as you want. You can mix up your menu to keep things interesting. There are a lot of healthy recipes available online that you can choose from. Create your own compilation of recipes and use these as a reference when planning your meals each week.

- **You save money**

  Again, meal planning helps you save a lot of money which you would have otherwise spent on prepared, packaged, processed, and unhealthy meals. You can save money by purchasing fresh and raw ingredients. You can also save money by limiting the number of times you dine out. This particular reason is why more and more people are becoming interested in meal planning. Who doesn't want to save money, right?

Tips for Meal Planning

As you can see, meal planning is highly beneficial. But if you don't know how to do this, you may feel overwhelmed. Just like any new skill or concept, you need to learn more about meal planning before you start doing it. Also, you should keep practicing meal planning to get better at it. Here are some pointers to start you off:

- **Plan your meals**

This is an obvious one. The first step in meal planning is the planning itself. Before you go shopping for ingredients, take time to sit down and think about what meals you want to eat for the week. To make it easier and more organized, have two lists with you. One for the meals and the other for the ingredients you need.

After completing these lists, check your kitchen or pantry compared to the list of ingredients you made. You may discover that you already have some of the ingredients you've written down. In this case, you can cross these items off your list, so you don't purchase them again.

- **Organize your recipes**

First, you have to search for recipes. A simple Google search will provide you with countless options. If you want to narrow down the options, choose the right keywords. For instance, if you want to look for easy-to-prepare breakfast recipes, use these keywords for your search or if you only want recipes which use plant-based ingredients, then use those keywords. When it comes to searching for recipes online, you have to be as specific as possible if you want to find something in particular.

After you've printed out all the recipes you find interesting, it's time to organize them. Purchase a binder or a clear book to store all these recipes. That way, you can refer to this file every time you sit down to plan your meals. As time goes by, you can keep looking for and adding new recipes to this book allowing you to mix and match your meals every week.

- **Check for leftovers**

  Before you sit down to plan your meals, check your refrigerator for any leftovers. You may have missed one or two of your meals from the previous week because you dined out or you were too tired to eat your meal before going to bed. No matter what your reason is, skipping meals leaves you with leftovers. In such a case, you can bump up these meals to the start of your week and only plan your meals for the rest of the days.

- **Plan strategically**

  While thinking about your meals, try to think of dishes which share the same ingredients. That way, you don't have to purchase too many ingredients at one time. This also makes it easier to prepare your meals when you only have a few ingredients for different kinds of dishes.

- **Consider making extra**

  The great thing about meal planning is that you can create as many meals as you want when it's time to cook. Another great tip is to make extra and store this in the freezer. That way, if you're not in the mood for the food you planned for a certain day, you have other options. Then you can simply bump up those meals you skipped for another day or for the next week. Just make sure that the meals you bump up to other days don't spoil easily so they won't go to waste.

- **Be flexible**

  Finally, don't take your meal planning too seriously. Allow yourself to have "cheat days" occasionally, especially when you're really craving something. The more you restrict yourself, the more you will feel negatively towards this new change you're trying to implement in your life. Remember to go easy on yourself and give yourself a break once in a while.

Tips for Grocery Shopping

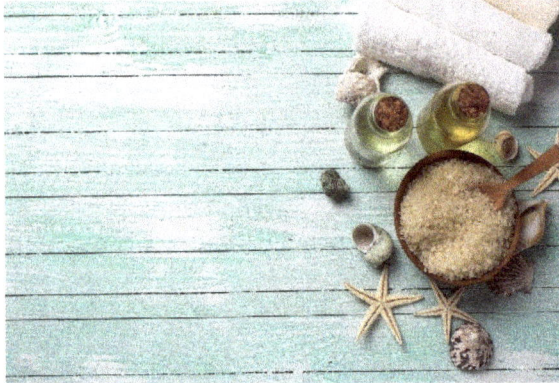

After planning your meals and the ingredients to use for those meals, it's time to hit the grocery store. Even before you start meal planning, it's a good idea to visit the local supermarkets, grocery stores, convenience stores, and farmer's markets to see what they have to offer. That way, you know whether you can make the recipes you've found online or if you can substitute some of the ingredients with the available options. This time, let's look at some valuable grocery shopping tips for you to keep in mind:

- **Always bring your shopping list with you**

  The moment you set foot into the supermarket, you will be faced with seemingly endless choices of food items, from fresh produce to snack items. It's easy to get overwhelmed in supermarkets and it's also easy to start buying impulsively, especially when you don't have a shopping list.

  If you recall our first tip for meal planning, it involves creating a list of ingredients you need for the meals you will be cooking. Since you've already made the list, make sure that you bring it with you when you go shopping. That way, you know exactly what to buy so you won't have to go to the other aisles that don't contain what you need.

- **Give yourself some options**

When you create your list of ingredients, it's also a good idea to give yourself other options in case the ingredients you need aren't available. This saves you a lot of time when you're unable to find the food items you need for your planned dishes. You can check the recipes to see possible substitutes for ingredients and note these down on your shopping list too.

- **Shopping for different food items**

If you aren't easily tempted and you enjoy going around the entire supermarket, there's nothing wrong with that. Even though you have a list, going around the supermarket gives you an idea or even inspiration for the meals you can plan for the next week. Here are some shopping tips for the different types of food items you may find in the supermarket:

  o When searching for fresh produce, choose different colors. These colors indicate the nutrient content of fruits and vegetables.
  o For pasta, bread, and cereals, go for the ones that are made from whole grains.
  o If you plan to continue eating fish, poultry, and meat, make sure to choose fresh fish, skinless poultry, and lean cuts of meat.
  o For dairy products, go for unflavored varieties, especially for milk and yogurt products.
  o Frozen foods are great, especially for times when you need to prepare a quick meal, as long as you don't rely on them too much.

o   Dried and canned foods are alright too as long as you choose products that don't contain high amounts of sugars, sodium, and artificial ingredients.

Chapter 6:
Believe in Yourself to Reach Your Goals

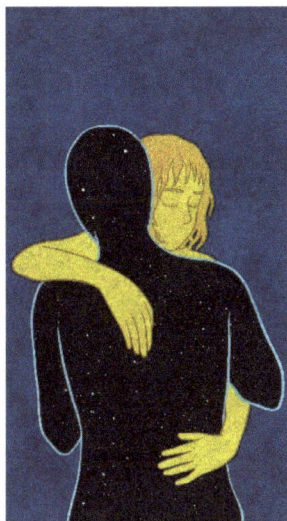

Loving your body goes beyond the physical aspect. This means that you can only truly love the skin you're in when you learn how to believe in yourself as well. Believing in yourself is an important aspect of reaching your goals. However, one thing you need to have in order to do this is the right motivation. Without motivation, you won't be able to keep going.

Too often, people give up on their quest for self-improvement because they lose their motivation. If you don't want to be one of these people, then you must actively look for ways to inspire intrinsic motivation. This type of motivation is far more powerful than the motivation you get from external rewards. Consider these statements when you're feeling unmotivated, stuck, or unwilling to push through with your plans:

- Find something that motivates you no matter what the activity may be.
- Focus on your goals and on the actionable steps which you have made for yourself.
- Change up your routine once in a while so you don't end up getting bored with it.
- Make things fun for yourself so you don't see the steps in your plans as chores or challenges.
- Write down your plans to serve as a physical reminder of what needs to be done.
- Find support from those closest to you in order to stay motivated.
- Reward yourself occasionally, especially after overcoming something particularly challenging.
- Allow yourself to make mistakes and learn from them.

If you keep all these tips in mind, you will find it a lot easier to believe in yourself and stay motivated throughout your journey, and when you start seeing positive changes in your life it will keep you more inspired to keep going. Positivity is important, especially when you're trying to improve your life.

Self-Confidence and Motivation

Motivation is a basic part of our lives. It's powerful enough to influence how and when we perform the tasks we need to do. Motivation is a hypothetical construct utilized in order to describe the external and internal forces that create the direction, intensity, persistence, and initiation of behavior.

Motivation can either be extrinsic or intrinsic depending on where the reward comes from. In general, people who depend on extrinsic motivation aren't as successful in reaching their goals compared to those who depend on intrinsic motivation. Still, extrinsic motivation can have powerful effects on a person, especially at the beginning of their journey.

Self-confidence is one factor that drives motivation. It can either hinder or help a person's performance depending on how much self-confidence the person has and what the task requires. Self-confidence is a person's belief in his own capacity to plan and organize actionable steps needed to produce specific results.

So, how are these related?

A person who has poor self-confidence may find it difficult to motivate themselves to achieve their goals. In fact, they might not even have the confidence to decide to improve their life. People without self-confidence, those who feel broken or defeated might not have the willingness to take that all-important first step.

When you look at it this way, how would such people be able to find the motivation to make their lives better when they don't even think that they can do anything right? If you feel that you lack self-confidence, this should be the first thing you work on even before you start learning to love your body.

Learn more about yourself, what you're good at, and what your strengths are. Doing this will help make you feel better about yourself, thus increasing your self-confidence. Also, you should spend more time with people who love and appreciate you. Think of them as your support system. Having a strong support system goes a long way in terms of building self-confidence. And when you feel like your self-confidence has improved, then you can start looking for ways to improve the other aspects of yourself.

How to Improve Your Self-Confidence

We all need self-confidence in order to succeed. If this is one of your weaknesses, then it's time to start improving yourself. Even if you grew up without self-confidence, there is still hope for you.

Self-confidence isn't something you're born with, it's something which you build. Although it would have been better if you grew up with self-confidence, you must work with what you have right now. So, if you're struggling with this, here are some ways to help you build your self-confidence:

- **Practice self-awareness**

  Self-awareness is the basis of self-confidence. Often though, this is overlooked. You cannot take action unless you know yourself and who you really are at your very core. It's important for you to understand all your strengths, weaknesses, dreams, and desires. The more self-aware you are, the more you will be able to build your self-confidence. Here are some self-awareness exercises to try:

  - Take some time for yourself in a room with no distractions. Close your eyes and try to see your life's story through the eyes of those around you. As you do this, try to see how your experiences have molded and influenced who you have become as a person.
  - Start a conversation with your family and your closest friends. Ask them what they think your strengths are as well as what you need to improve on. Ensure them that you're totally open to constructive criticism and that you won't feel bad when they tell you about your weaknesses.
  - Try mindful meditation. This is an excellent way to become more aware of your body, your thoughts, and your feelings.

- **Do things that make you happy**

  When you enjoy the things you do, you feel more confident in doing them. Therefore, if you choose to do things that make you happy, the more it will help build your self-confidence. This is why it's a good idea to pair exercising with activities you enjoy such as listening to music and watching TV.

Even cooking can become a more enjoyable activity while you listen to your favorite tunes. Over time, you won't even notice that you're getting better at the things you're doing because you're having so much fun. Then when you realize that you've improved without realizing it, it will be a huge confidence booster for you.

- **Practice positive visualization and self-talk**

  Negativity has a huge impact on your self-confidence. When you hear other people say mean or derogatory things about you all the time, you might start believing them. When you start internalizing the bad thoughts, words, and actions of those around you, your self-confidence starts to plummet.

  To combat this, you should try practicing positive visualization and self-talk. Positive visualization involves thinking of situations where you succeed. For instance, you can try visualizing yourself already achieving the goals you've set. Try to picture how you look, feel, act, and so on. The more you visualize all these things, the more your subconscious starts working to achieve them.

  The same thing goes for positive self-talk. Keep reminding yourself of your strengths and how well you are progressing. The more you encourage yourself, the more confident you will become in your capabilities. Combine these two and you'll start seeing see huge changes in your life.

- **Give journaling a try**

  Starting and maintaining a journal is an excellent way to build your self-confidence. In your journal, you can write down anything that makes you feel good. You can write down your goals, dreams, strengths, and all the other good things in your life. You can also write down the good things you want to have in your life and how you plan to achieve them.

  Maintaining a journal is both cathartic and healthy. Write down any achievements you've made, any breakthroughs, and any challenges. Take some time at the end of each day to add an entry into your journal. This helps build your self-confidence because you're able to see how well you are progressing and how much your life has improved compared to when you started.

- **Don't compare yourself to other people**

  If you want to improve your self-confidence, this is something you should stop *right now*. Keep reminding yourself that you're a unique individual so you should never compare yourself with others. Picture this: you feel insecure about your body and you wish you could change. Now, what do you think will happen when you keep comparing yourself to someone who you think has the "perfect body." Most likely, you'll end up wallowing in self-pity.

  This is a dangerous situation because there is a high likelihood that you would just give up and accept defeat. Rather than comparing yourself to others, think about all your capabilities as well as the things you can do to improve your body or whatever it is you want to improve.

- **Be compassionate to yourself**

   Finally, learn how to be more compassionate to yourself. The kinder you are to yourself, the more you will have the confidence to tackle tasks head-on. By contrast, the harder you are on yourself, the more likely you'll feel like you cannot really make a difference in your life. So, which situation seems more appealing to you?

Chapter 7:
A Day in the Life of Self-love

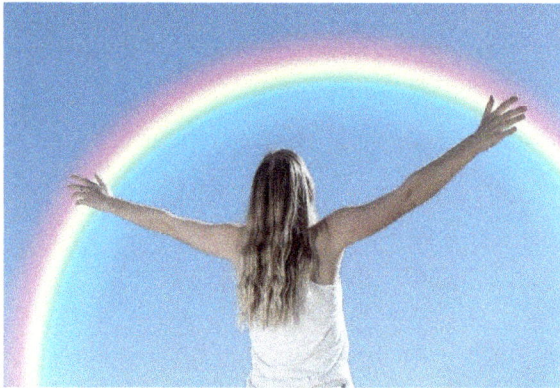

By now you have more than enough information to help you learn how to truly love your body. From everything we've discussed so far, you may notice that it's all about you. That's because learning to love your body also means learning more about yourself.

Caring for your emotional health is just as essential as caring for your physical health. Even though you're able to eat well and exercise regularly, if you ignore your emotional health, you won't be able to truly accept and appreciate all that you are. As a matter of fact, when your emotional health is suffering, you might start experiencing physical symptoms such as chest pains, ulcers, high blood pressure, and more. On the other hand, when you are emotionally stable, you will find it a lot easier to deal with challenges from the small issues to the large events that happen in your life.

Have you ever wondered how you can truly love your body and everything else about yourself? This is a process that doesn't happen overnight. It takes a lot of time, effort, patience, and compassion in order to reach a place where you can genuinely say that you love and accept yourself for who you are. Here are some ways to help you achieve this:

- **Strengthen your support system**

  If you want to bring more positivity into your life, you need a strong support system. Your support system is composed of the people who love you, accept you, and will be there for you in times of doubt and tribulation. Keep in touch with these people to ensure that your relationships don't fade away.

- **Learn how to lessen your fears**

  The best way to do this is to learn more about them. For instance, if you're suffering from a medical condition and you're afraid of how this might affect your life, try to learn as much as you can about it both from your doctor and your own research. The more you learn, the less you'll fear what may happen next because you're prepared for it.

- **Keep moving to lessen your anxiety and improve your mood**

  Remaining physically active is important, especially when you find activities that you actually enjoy. We've gone through the physical and mental benefits of physical activity. But there are social and emotional benefits to this too. When you keep moving, this helps lessen your anxiety and gives your mood a much-needed boost.

- **Have sex!**

  Speaking of enjoyable activities, having sex is an excellent example. When you have sex with someone you love and trust, this level of intimacy helps build your self-worth and your confidence. It makes you feel good physically and it also improves your emotional health.

- **Invest in a new hobby or skill**

  Learning new things or starting new hobbies can improve your life. Investing time in learning a new skill or practicing a new hobby makes you feel fulfilled. The more you practice, the more enjoyable these skills or hobbies will be. Then you'll start seeing a change in your self-confidence as well as how you perceive yourself.

- **Practice yoga or meditation**

  These activities are also highly beneficial in terms of learning self-love. They build your self-awareness, which allows you to focus on your thoughts, feelings, and needs. Aside from this, yoga and meditation are also excellent stress relievers.

- **Avoid overextending yourself**

  It's important for you to learn how to say "no" once in a while, especially when you really can't deal with everything. There's nothing wrong with declining requests or invitations, just make sure to do this in a polite and positive way. Don't assume that people will have ill feelings towards you if you don't say "yes" to them each and every time.

  As long as you explain why you have to decline, chances are they will understand your situation and accept your rejection without feeling bad. Give others a chance so you don't end up overextending yourself.

- **Learn how to manage your time properly**

  Often, you may forget to focus on or prioritize yourself because you always feel like there's not enough time to get everything done. This is especially true when you have a day job and it's particularly stressful. To ease your situation, try to learn how to manage your time better. Come up with a schedule that allows you to take care of yourself while still being able to do all the other important things assigned to you.

A Sample Schedule Which Promotes Self-love

Self-love doesn't have to be just a dream. As you can see, there are several ways for you to nurture love and acceptance for yourself. So, what does a day in the life of self-love look like? Here's a sample schedule/routine which promotes self-love:

- Wake up early so you don't have to rush through your morning.
- Go outside for about 5 minutes or so to breathe in the fresh air, experience the warmth of the morning sun, and just appreciate the moment.
- Take some time to stretch or meditate for about 10 minutes. You may also use this time to practice mindfulness exercises instead of meditation or stretching.
- Heat up the breakfast you had prepared and stored in the refrigerator for this day.
- Get ready for work. Don't forget to bring your lunch for this day!
- Walk to work if it's not that far. If you need to drive, park your car far from your building so you can still walk from your parking space to your workplace.
- Check all the tasks you need to accomplish for the day. Make a list of all these tasks and arrange them by the level of importance.
- Occasionally, get up and walk around the office. Don't forget to hydrate yourself. You may also strike up conversations with your colleagues once in a while to break the monotony.

- Have lunch. Heat up the packed meal you've brought with you. Converse with your workmates while eating. Share stories, experiences, and laughs.
- Go back to work. Continue with the list of tasks you created when you came in.
- Clock out and go home.
- Have dinner with your family.
- Start your wind-down or bedtime routine.
- Go to sleep at a reasonable hour.

This is a sample schedule you could adopt. As you can see, a lot of the activities involve ways on how you can promote self-love. From eating healthy meals, staying hydrated, interacting with others, having physical activity, and more. There are plenty of ways to deal with your daily life while still taking care of yourself.

You can come up with your own schedule as well and it doesn't have to be the same each day. Make adjustments if you have to and change your routine up to keep things interesting.

A Sample Meal Plan to Go with Your Day

Now that you have a better idea of a schedule you can work with, let's look at a sample meal plan to go with the previous sample schedule. Remember that you would have already prepared all your meals even before the week started. This makes it easier for you to eat regularly since all you have to do is heat up the meals you've planned and prepared. Here's a sample meal plan for you:

- **Breakfast:**

    Pancakes with cream cheese, butter, and syrup (sugar-free)

    Coffee, heavy cream, and sweetener (no carb)

    Breakfast sausage (sugar-free) or bacon

- **Lunch**

  Pancakes with cream cheese this time with ham, cheese, mayonnaise, and spinach or arugula.

- **Snacks**

  2-3 pieces of string cheese or half an avocado sprinkled with salt and pepper

- **Dinner**

  Buffalo wings with blue cheese dressing (sugar-free)

  Celery sticks

- **Dessert (optional)**

  1 serving of chocolate truffles or chocolate mousse

This is just a sample meal plan. The meals you have each day would depend on what kind of diet you have chosen and what you have planned for the week.

Conclusion

It's Time to Start Changing Your Life!

There you go! A brief but comprehensive guide to help you learn how to love your body and everything else about you. In this book, we have gone through some clever secrets to help you reinvent your life, change your body, and improve your mind. As you may have noticed, all the things we have gone through are focused on you. How you can start your journey, how you can keep yourself motivated, and how you can learn to love and accept who you are as well as the body you have.

Always remember that you can do this! As long as you set goals, make plans, and do whatever it takes to build your self-confidence and self-worth. Start off small and gradually work your way towards your goals. The more you're able to achieve your short-term goals, the more inspired you will be. And if you stick with it, you'll see that your love for your body and yourself has grown significantly since you began this journey of self-improvement. Good luck!

Bibliography

5 steps to start a fitness program. (2018). Retrieved from
https://www.mayoclinic.org/healthy-lifestyle/fitness/in-
depth/fitness/art-20048269

5 Proven Ways to Build Self Confidence and Take Life Head On -
Fearless Motivation. (2018). Retrieved from
https://www.fearlessmotivation.com/2017/08/28/9318/

10 Simple Tricks to Make You a Meal Planning Genius. (2016).
Retrieved from https://www.lifeasastraw-
berry.com/meal-planning-genius/

10 TIPS TO MOTIVATE YOURSELF TO LIVE A HEALTHY
LIFESTYLE. (2018). Retrieved from http://promis-
eorpay.com/blog/10-tips-to-motivate-yourself-to-live-a-
healthy-lifestyle/

15 Helpful Tips to Stop Binge Eating. (2019). Retrieved from
https://www.healthline.com/nutrition/how-to-stop-
binge-eating#section15

23 Effective Ways to Stop Overeating. (2019). Retrieved from
https://www.healthline.com/nutrition/how-to-stop-over-
eating

Cheek, E. The Relationship Between Motivation, Self- Confidence and Anxiety - The UK's leading Sports Psychology
Website. (2019). Retrieved from https://believeper-
form.com/performance/the-relationship-between-moti-
vation-self-confidence-and-anxiety/

Crichton-Stuart, C. The top 10 benefits of eating healthy. (2018). Retrieved from https://www.medicalnewstoday.com/articles/322268.php

Dave, C. Mental And Physical Benefits Of Exercise. (2016). Retrieved from https://www.huffpost.com/entry/mental-and-physical-benefits-of-exercise_n_57d6341be4b0f831f70722f8

Davis, T. Self-Care: 12 Ways to Take Better Care of Yourself. (2018). Retrieved from https://www.psychologytoday.com/us/blog/click-here-happiness/201812/self-care-12-ways-take-better-care-yourself

McCarthy, M. How Journaling Can Boost Your Self-Confidence. (2019). Retrieved from https://www.mindbodygreen.com/0-5139/How-Journaling-Can-Boost-Your-SelfConfidence.html

Morin, A. 5 Ways to Start Boosting Your Self-Confidence Today. (2019). Retrieved from https://www.verywellmind.com/how-to-boost-your-self-confidence-4163098

Orenstein, B. 10 Ways to Boost Your Emotional Health Through Improving Your Self-Esteem. (2017). Retrieved from https://www.everydayhealth.com/emotional-health/10-ways-to-boost-emotional-health.aspx

Physical Activity: Keeping Motivated | Nutrition Australia. (2019). Retrieved from http://www.nutritionaustralia.org/national/resource/physical-activity-keeping-motivated

Rosenberg, M. The Do's and Don'ts of Self-Care | Bella Grace Magazine. (2019). Retrieved from https://bellagracemagazine.com/blog/the-dos-and-donts-of-self-care/

Self-esteem and Motivation - Maslow's Hierarchy of Needs. (2017). Retrieved from https://www.psychology-noteshq.com/maslowhierarchyofneeds/

The 4 Fallacies of Undereating - and How to Overcome This Negative Thinking - Leanness Lifestyle University. (2019). Retrieved from https://lluniversity.com/the-4-fallacies-of-undereating-and-how-to-overcome-this-negative-thinking/

The Dos and Don'ts of Self-Care - College Fashion. (2018). Retrieved from https://www.collegefashion.net/college-life/self-care-dos-and-donts/

The Importance of Meal Planning: 3 Reasons to Meal Plan Weekly. (2019). Retrieved from https://projectmeal-plan.com/importance-of-meal-planning/

The Top 10 Home Cooking Health Benefits. (2016). Retrieved from https://www.healthfitnessrevolution.com/top-10-health-benefits-cooking-home/

Valente, L. 7 Tips for Clean Eating. (2019). Retrieved from http://www.eatingwell.com/article/78846/7-tips-for-clean-eating/

Wagner, G. 25 Ways to Make Time for Fitness. (2011). Retrieved from https://experiencelife.com/article/25-ways-to-make-time-for-fitness/

Zelman, K. 10 Tips for Healthy Grocery Shopping. (2019). Retrieved from https://www.webmd.com/food-recipes/features/10-tips-for-healthy-grocery-shopping#1

Zeratsky, K. Clean eating is more than washing your hands. (2019). Retrieved from https://www.mayo-clinic.org/healthy-lifestyle/nutrition-and-healthy-eating/expert-answers/clean-eating/faq-20336262

www.ingramcontent.com/pod-product-compliance
Lightning Source LLC
Chambersburg PA
CBHW041218030426

42336CB00023B/3381